Are Superfoods Healthy?

The Benefits of Superfoods

By: Mark Wilson

PUBLISHERS NOTES

Disclaimer

This publication is intended to provide helpful and informative material. It is not intended to diagnose, treat, cure, or prevent any health problem or condition, nor is intended to replace the advice of a physician. No action should be taken solely on the contents of this book. Always consult your physician or qualified health-care professional on any matters regarding your health and before adopting any suggestions in this book or drawing inferences from it.

The author and publisher specifically disclaim all responsibility for any liability, loss or risk, personal or otherwise, which is incurred as a consequence, directly or indirectly, from the use or application of any contents of this book.

Any and all product names referenced within this book are the trademarks of their respective owners. None of these owners have sponsored, authorized, endorsed, or approved this book.

Always read all information provided by the manufacturers' product labels before using their products. The author and publisher are not responsible for claims made by manufacturers.

Paperback Edition

Manufactured in the United States of America

DEDICATION

This book is dedicated to all the parents who made us eat our vegetables on a daily basis. I would also like to thank my mentor Jack, who guided me through the research process and was always there to support me when I was ready to give up.

Table of Contents

Publishers Notes 2

Dedication 3

Chapter 1- What Are Superfoods? 5

Chapter 2- How Superfoods Benefit The Body 11

Chapter 3- How The Top 10 Superfoods Benefit The Body 16

Chapter 4- Superfoods That Help To Burn Fat 22

Chapter 5- Superfoods That Help With Weight Loss   27

Chapter 6- Superfoods That Help To Build Muscle 32

Chapter 7- Superfoods- Frequently Asked Questions   37

About The Author 42

Chapter 1 - What Are Superfoods?

When one thinks of the term "Superfoods", they can be forgiven for getting a visual image of Superman or perhaps the Avengers going out to grab a super-sized burger and fries. After all, doesn't "superfoods" refer to heaping portions of delicious foods that aren't so good for you? Actually, our caped pals should be sitting down to a meal including Superfoods at the S.H.I.E.L.D. or the Fortress of Solitude, and not because they can afford those calories. Superfoods may not be what they or you think they are.

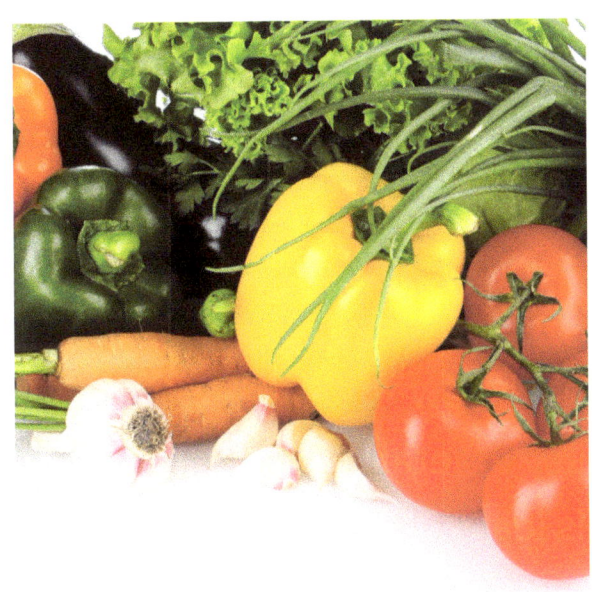

"Superfoods" refers to a group that's represented across the food spectrum; largely fruits and vegetables, but meat, fish, and dairy are represented here as well. We all remember from nutrition class in school that many different kinds of food provide vital nutrients and vitamins essential to good health, but "superfoods"

are, super, for yet another reason. They have been proven to provide health benefits well beyond just a few vitamins.

Apples, for example, are wonderful sources of Vitamin C. It doesn't matter which variety you munch on; eating just one apple a day will provide you with a quarter of the Vitamin C you should have to get through your day. And not just that, an apple a day also helps keep your digestive system on track, and can lower your cholesterol levels. And of course, keeps the doctor away. See, those old sayings aren't just catchy! So what other fruits or vegetables should you be incorporating into your daily diet?

Fruits/Vegetables

Spinach

Your mother and Popeye were right. This classic "eat it, it's good for you veggie" has now been determined to be the most nutritious of not just vegetables, but all foods. Iron is among the many nutrients this leafy plant contains, in addition to a veritable alphabet of vitamins, primary among them, vitamins C, F, K, and B.

Broccoli

Yes, you have to eat this one, too. This vegetable is another good source of Vitamin C and many nutrients, and has been proven to have anti-cancer properties, and help prevent macular degeneration. Cook or munch on 5 to 7 broccoli florets (heads and stems) raw to get the full benefit of this vegetable.

Kale

This lettuce-like plant contains no fat, but lots of fiber, which makes it a perfect food for digestive tract issues. Kale also contains anti-inflammatory properties, making it a good food choice for those suffering from auto-immune disorders, such as asthma and arthritis.

Avocados

Break out the dip! The "butter pear", once looked at as an exotic, expensive resident of the produce aisle got its nickname because it contains a high amount of fat. Wait! Don't run away! We indeed need a certain degree of fat in our diets, and not only does the avocado contain "good fat", this beneficial fat assists our body's "good" cholesterol. In other words, it helps keep our cholesterol at proper levels. This fruit is also a good source of fiber, potassium, and Vitamins C and K.

Blueberries

This tasty little fruit has a number of health benefits. Not only does it contain the ever popular Vitamin C, the blueberry has anti-cancer and anti-diabetes properties, and research has shown that it may slow down the aging of nerve cells.

Meat and Fish

Beef

What! This must be a typo! After all, didn't decades of eating those big, juicy steaks result in plenty of heart attacks? It is true that one must be more cautious in consuming these particular superfoods, but there are a number of health benefits to be derived for the prudent consumer. Beef underwent a health backlash for a number of years, but lean cuts of red meat can provide great benefits to muscle and hair health, as well as heart health. Just steer clear of fatty cuts of it. One way to do so would be to consume beef from North America's native cow, the bison. Once almost extinct in this country, today it flourishes not only on the prairie, but as livestock on ranches. Its meat is prepared in the same way as "traditional" beef, and has considerably less fat.

Fish

Consumers have known for a while now about the health properties of the high levels of Omega-3 found in fish oil. It is beneficial in combatting both heart disease and arthritis. Salmon, tuna, and mackerel are all good choices here; just make sure they come from mercury-free sources.

Dairy

Yogurt

The superhero of dairy superfoods, yogurt is a great source of calcium, protein, and potassium while containing less lactose than other products, making it great for the digestive system, too.

Skim Milk

Skim milk has all the benefits of other dairy products, plus fewer calories, too.

Superfood Super Easy Recipe

Easy Avocado Dip

Things you'll need:

- 4 large dark green avocados
- Vegetable parker
- Mixing bowl
- Table spoon
- 1/2 cup salsa
- Potato masher
- Garlic salt
- Lemon juice

Instructions:

- Pare and cut each avocado lengthwise into two sections.
- Use tablespoon to spoon the pulp, or meat, from each avocado into the mixing bowl.

- Use the potato masher to cream the pulp to the desired consistency.
- Add and stir in the salsa.
- Add garlic salt by the pinch for additional flavoring.
- And a squeeze or two of lemon juice to prevent browning. Chill and serve.

CHAPTER 2 - HOW SUPERFOODS BENEFIT THE BODY

Superfoods have been on the tip of the tongues of those who have made a commitment to better eating and living. This is because there are truly some foods that are simply super for the body. Each has the ability to provide the body with the right mix of nutrients that is required. In fact, many superfoods have been associated with healing and improving body functionality, as these foods are comprised of the right mix of vitamins, minerals and antioxidants. To better understand why and how these superfoods are beneficial it is best to understand which superfoods hold the most promise for better well-being.

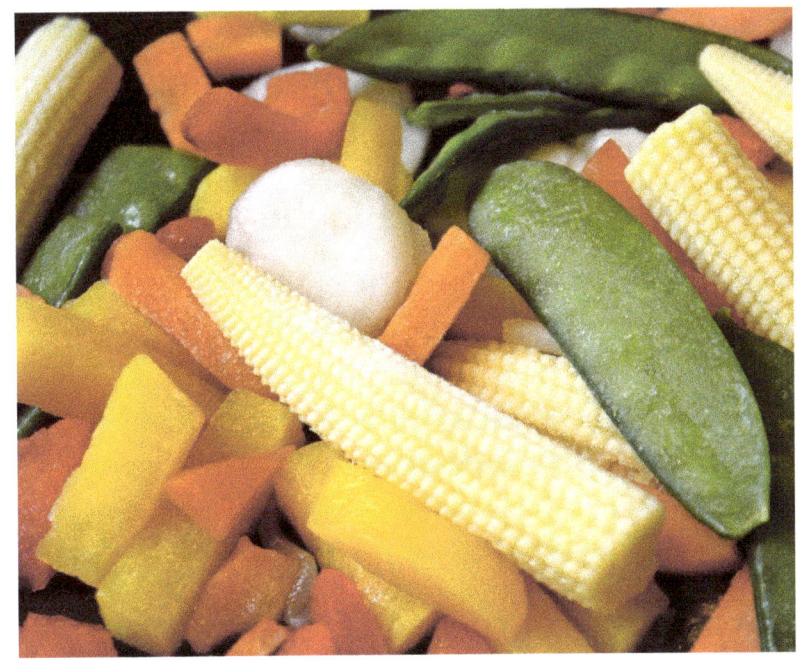

Sardines

Once thought of as something grandparents ate because they were shelf stable during the depression era, research has come to show that sardines are in fact a superfood. The main reason these rank high as a superfood is the high amount of Omega-3 fat that is found within each of these tiny fish. They are also high in both calcium and protein which makes them a low cost superfood that does various parts of the body good. From brain functions, to bone density, sardines are truly a beneficial food.

Blueberries

Blueberries have been touted as a superfood for years as they have so many benefits and they appeal to just about everyone. Blueberries have naturally occurring flavonoids which just happen to be a beneficial element for brain function. In addition, this one superfood also is helpful in keeping kidneys clean, staving off cancer cell growth and improving blood flow. There have also been numerous studies touting memory improvement when one consumes blueberries regularly. Blueberries can be eaten raw, cooked or even brewed as tea since the benefits come through regardless of how those deep dark berries are served.

Spinach

Once a cringe worthy food that many misunderstood, spinach has proven to be tasty when served properly and highly beneficial to the body. The high levels of beta carotene, Vitamin C, Vitamin K and iron make this one food almost a multi-vitamin that comes in plant form. As mentioned in chapter 1, the routine consumption of spinach helps boost the immune system through the high antioxidant properties of the spinach and helps make bones stronger, teeth healthier, muscles more flexible and even promotes better hair and skin. The benefits of spinach seem almost too many to list as this superfood is truly a star in its own right. It is best to eat raw or par boiled spinach as this helps preserve the bulk of the nutrients that make this a superfood.

Deep and Dark Chocolate

One of the more surprising superfoods out there is none other than everyone's favorite vice and that is none other than chocolate. Dark chocolate is the true superfood and not the standard issue and over processed candy bars found in grocery stores at the checkout area. Dark chocolate is high in pure cacao and that is where the superfood status comes in to play. Flavonoids and antioxidants are found naturally in cacao and that can go a long way in supporting the body. It has been proven that dark chocolate can lower blood pressure, increase blood vessel flow, reduce cholesterol and even boost moods. This again is why this is a superfood, as it does various things for various parts of the body all at the same time.

Plenty of Other Choices

There are ample other superfoods out there that can truly make a difference in how one looks and feels. Some superfoods are more surprising than others such as pistachio nuts and sweet red bell peppers. The key to incorporating superfoods into ones daily diet is to look into those nutritional qualities of all the foods one eats. Superfoods are labeled as such due to their natural ability to provide more than one beneficial quality that the human body craves, needs, wants and can use for creating a better body in general. Once one gets the hang of figuring out how to rank and rate foods, they will find plenty of superfoods exist and that makes it much easier to get them added to daily life through diet.

Superfoods have been gaining quite a following as people have been eating more clean and green. This has caused people to be much more educated in terms of the foods they eat and this is why superfoods have garnered so much attention. The attention is well deserved because who would have thought that eating blueberries every day could in fact reverse some serious health issues, taste great and make a body stronger in ways one may have never even imagined. That is why superfoods are worth a top spot in the diet of everyone as they do so much for the body that it would be hard to find a superfood that did not benefit one in any manner.

The transition to better living really can be driven by a change in diet. This is because the body truly does function from the inside out and when the right superfoods are fed to the body it uses those foods for all that they offer. This in turn leads to a strong body and to a better quality of life. The fact that one can replicate some healing qualities once only found through modern medicine or medical intervention is an amazing thing to behold. Those who have found that eating superfoods on a routine basis has transitioned their quality of life will attest to the fact that superfoods really are super foods to eat, drink and simply enjoy.

CHAPTER 3- HOW THE TOP 10 SUPERFOODS BENEFIT THE BODY

I usually eat approximately 1lb of organic butter per week, as this is an exceptional source of getting the nutrients that are needed for a wide range of bodily functions. When you are trying to keep a healthy body, it is essential that you consume healthy things. That old saying that you always heard when you were a child, "you are what you eat", is actually true. If you eat unhealthy foods, you will be unhealthy. If you eat healthy foods, you will be healthy.

Over the past few years, the word "superfood" has become very popular. A superfood is a food item that has all of the essential vitamins and nutrients that the body needs in order to be healthy. Many processed-food companies claim that their products contain these superfoods. This is untrue. When a food is processed, it loses most of its vitamins and nutrients during processing. These foods may have been superfoods before being processed, however, once the food is processed, it is no longer considered to be a superfood. Superfoods are basically pure organic foods. They are not processed and contain no preservatives. There are many foods that can be categorized as superfoods. Below is a list of the top 10 most important superfoods that your body needs in order to stay in shape.

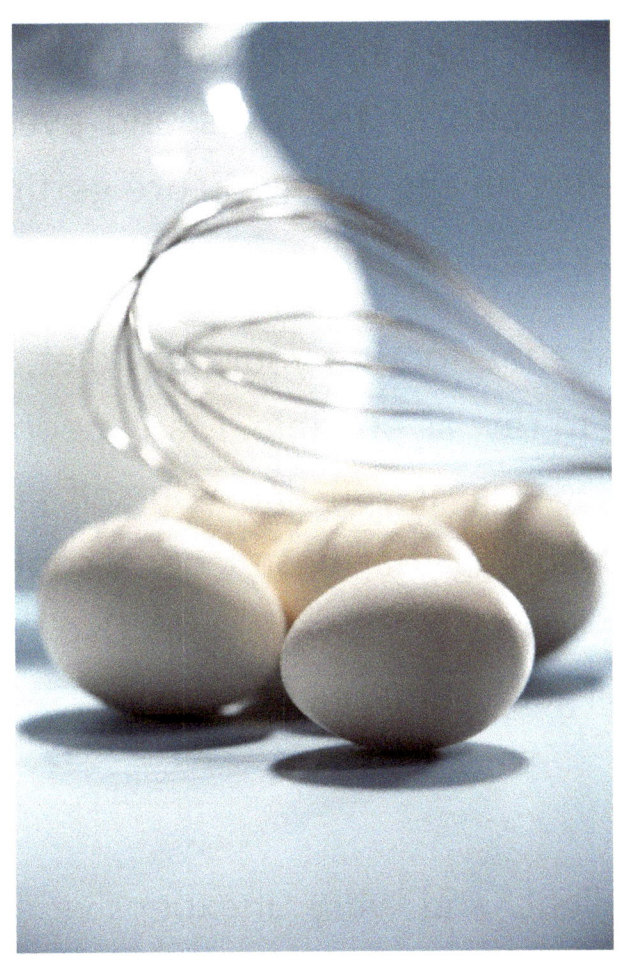

Free-Range Eggs

Free range eggs are considered to be a superfood because just one egg contains everything that your body needs to be healthy. Eggs have the highest quality protein that you can find in any food. Protein is necessary to build, maintain, and repair body tissues such as muscles, internal organs, and the skin. This protein also boosts your immune system and keeps your hormones balanced. Eggs contain nine essential amino acids; there are not many foods that do. Eggs also contain choline. Choline is necessary for your brain and nervous system to keep them functioning properly. Choline is also beneficial to the cardiovascular system. Eggs also contain two of the components necessary for the health of the eyes and eyesight, lutein and zeaxanthin. By eating an egg daily, you are getting the amount of B12 that your body requires daily.

When you add this superfood to your daily diet, it is important to eat them as close to raw as possible. Many people cannot handle eating an uncooked egg. If you find yourself getting sick at the thought of eating an egg that hasn't been cooked, eating them poached or soft-boiled is a very effective way to eat this superfood and still get its amazing nutrients.

Kale

Kale is an excellent and very inexpensive superfood. It is responsible for keeping many of your body systems healthy. Kale contains properties which provide the body with calcium and Indole-3 which can help to protect against colon cancer and other ailments. It also contains vitamin D. From this vitamin D, you get lutein and zeaxanthin. As stated above, lutein and zeaxanthin are very beneficial to the eyes and can protect against macular degeneration. Kale is also an excellent source of iron.

Kale can be used in a variety of ways. Some people like to steam kale and have it as their vegetable with dinner. Some people put kale in a soup or in as stew. For those who enjoy juicing or making healthy shakes, kale is a common ingredient.

Avocado

Avocados are one of the best superfoods. This is because they have various essential nutrients which helps improve your health. Avocados contain fiber, potassium, vitamin E and many other vitamins. Avocados are an excellent source of healthy raw fat as well. Not only do avocados have the nutrients necessary to keep you healthy, they also help your body to absorb fat soluble nutrients.

Some people add avocados to their omelets at breakfast and into their salads at lunch. People who blend and juice often use avocados in their recipes.

Green Vegetable Juice

Many people take to their blenders to get their daily serving of superfoods. Juicing fresh green vegetables has many benefits. One reason why many people juice their green vegetables is to promote weight loss. Drinking green vegetable juice is a low calorie treat which can increase energy, thereby providing the additional energy that you need to get in a good workout. Because green vegetable juice is utilized by the body immediately, it can give you a feeling of instant energy.

Studies have shown that people who make green vegetable juice a part of their daily diet are 76% less likely to develop Alzheimer's disease.

Green vegetable juice will also keep you healthy when everyone around you seems to be sick because it boosts your immune system. The stronger your immune system is, the more difficult it is for viruses to invade your body.

Raw Organic Grass Fed Butter

Most people use butter daily. Whether it is on a piece of toast or over fresh steamed vegetables, butter is an important part of our daily diets. The best type of butter is raw organic grass fed butter. This butter is made from the milk of cows that are fed nothing but grass.

Raw organic grass fed butter contains vitamin A, vitamin D, vitamin E, and K2. These vitamins are necessary for a wide range of functions in the body. This type of butter also contains the healthy type of fat that your body needs, such as omega-3 and omega-6 fats. These are excellent for brain function and skin health.

These types of butter also contain a compound that is known for protecting the body from cancer, known as conjugated linoelic acid (CLA). CLA also helps to facilitate the body's muscle building process instead of storing fat.

Adding superfoods to your diet is very important and actually very simple. As long as you know what foods to add, you can be creative and use them in many different ways.

CHAPTER 4- SUPERFOODS THAT HELP TO BURN FAT

There are a number of foods with benefits such as antioxidants and even fat burning capabilities. Foods that burn fat work by causing physiological changes in the body. Body fat is controlled by things such as the regulation of blood glucose levels and insulin. Thermogenics heat the body resulting in calorie burning through an increase in heart rate. Eating the proper combination of super foods will aid you in the burning of fat naturally.

Oranges

There aren't a lot of calories in oranges and the fiber aids in the regulation of blood glucose levels which should lessen the concern over the naturally occurring sugars. Functioning is improved with the vitamin C contained in oranges and the sweetness will prevent you from grabbing sweets when you want a snack.

Tomatoes

Tomatoes can help with the loss of weight and keep it from returning. They are high in fiber and low in calories. A number of conditions and diseases can be improved by the antioxidants from lycopene found in tomatoes.

Oats

The insoluble fiber increases metabolism and the carbohydrates found in them aids in a longer lasting feeling of being full to prevent overeating when oats are included in the diet. Oats also contain minerals and antioxidants while aiding in the lowering of cholesterol levels. Using skim milk to make the oats or eating unflavored oatmeal instead of flavored oatmeal containing sugar and preservatives will aid in burning fat.

Spices/Herbs

Experimenting with seasonings can add a bit of excitement to otherwise boring foods when you are trying to lose weight while aiding in an increase of metabolism. Calories are burned with black pepper, energy levels increase with ginseng. The process that breaks up fat is aided by turmeric; digestion is aided by ginger and the metabolism gets a boost from mustard seed.

Garlic is an herb that helps to lower the levels of blood sugar in the body and helps to begin the body's heat producing process known as thermogenics. Unhealthy fats are released from the body as a result of the allicin contained in garlic.

Ginger is used in numerous dishes around the world, but its medical benefits are fairly unknown. It acts as an activator for metabolism and aids in regulation of the body's metabolic rate. The strong favor of ginger means that you can tone it down by using it as a tea with honey and lemon drops or sprinkling it on your food.

Cinnamon, a highly aromatic spice aids in the burning of fat by allowing glucose faster entry into the cells while reducing the amount of insulin that reaches them. It only takes a forth of a teaspoon to get fat burning results.

Sweet Potatoes

There are fewer calories in sweet potatoes than regular baked potatoes. Not only will you remain satisfied longer but they contain Vitamin B6, Vitamin C, potassium and fiber which are all good for you.

Apples

There are low amounts of fat, sodium and calories in apples while they contain fiber to help keep you full between meals and aid in digestion. Purchasing organic apples will allow you to leave the peels on them so you can get the nutrients contained in them as well.

Apple cider vinegar contains a number of minerals, vitamins and acetic acid allowing it to control hunger while decreasing the storage of fat and aiding with the body's pH balance.

Nuts

Peanuts, pecans, walnuts and almonds are all healthy, natural foods that can aid in burning fat whether eaten alone or as part of a meal. Almonds contain niacin which prevents bloating and helps the digestive track to function correctly. The healthy fat in nuts aids you in maintaining a full feeling longer which reduces the potential for snacks between meals.

Avocados

The monounsaturated fats contained in avocados help with heart health and also provide fiber to help with the digestive process. The fruit also contains anti-fungal and anti-bacterial properties to aid in keeping you healthy. Weight is balanced by the amino acid lecithin found in them. The hormones that cause fat to be stored are kept at a distance while the fruit works with hormones that promote the burning of fat.

Coconut

The entire coconut is full of nutrients whether it is the meat, coconut cream, milk or oil. The MCTs (medium chained triglycerides) found in coconuts are used as energy by the body which makes cooking with coconut oil better for you. The opportunity to store fat is reduced which increases the amount of fat that is burnt.

Beans and Legumes

The lower calories, high fiber and protein content of beans and legumes make replacing meat with them a good way to burn fat. Stored fat is reduced as a result of the fiber and lack of saturated fats. The protein content does mean that they should be avoided at night, or a walk taken after eating them.

Water

While technically not a food, water is essential to aiding the body in the fat burning process. It can satisfy hunger that has been confused with thirst as well as removing toxins from the body. Drinking water about fifteen minutes before eating will not only keep you from being thirsty but it will help to reduce the amount that you eat during the meal, automatically lowering the amount of calories that are consumed. Ridding the body of chemicals, fats and excess nutrients can be achieved by drinking between eight and ten glasses of water daily.

Incorporating these superfoods into the diet will aid in the burning of fat, resulting in weight loss and prevent weight gain.

CHAPTER 5- SUPERFOODS THAT HELP WITH WEIGHT LOSS

There is an undeniable new and lasting trend moving through the population. Health conscious individuals are always looking for ways to increase the nutrients in their diet because they know there are numerous benefits to living a healthy lifestyle that includes balanced eating and daily exercise. A good rule of thumb for beginners is to select the most brightly colored fruits and vegetables from the produce market because they contain the most antioxidants and offer the most beneficial rewards to the body and even to the mind.

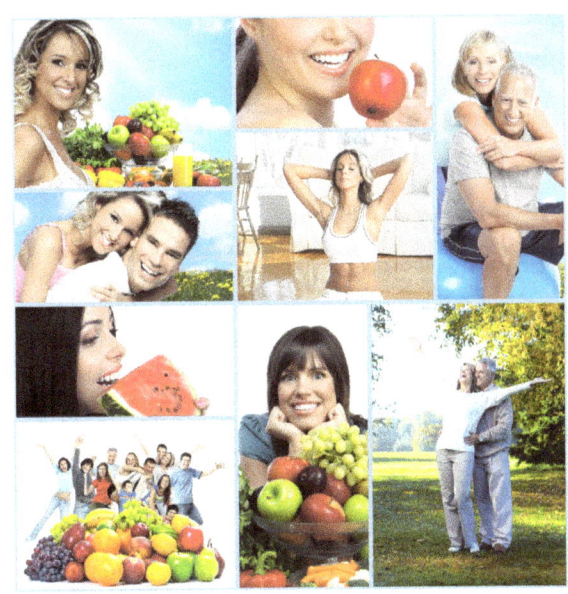

General Benefits to Healthy Eating

Medical professionals and researchers have spent decades trying to convince their patients to take better care of their overall health. For many people, this starts with drinking more water and eating less junk food that offers nothing but processed ingredients and empty calories that the body stores as additional fat supplies.

Eating habits, whether they are good ones or not, begin when people are very young so it can be difficult to change these habits once they are engrained in the psyche. People tend to say they do not like a food before they even try it because they have trained their body to accept certain foods and avoid others. This challenge can be overcome quite simply by slowly adding in new healthy foods while simultaneously reducing the amount and types of harmful foods in the diet. Over a relatively brief period the taste buds will accept these delicious new foods and the body will even begin to crave them instead of sweet treats and other carbohydrate gorged snacks.

Chronic health conditions such as high cholesterol, high blood pressure and heart disease can cause significant damage to the internal organs over time. Diabetes is quickly growing to become the number one killer of children and adults in many nations because of poor eating habits and lack of exercise. Many of those effects can be reduced or even reversed simply by eating a healthy diet rich in vitamins, minerals, essential fatty acids, fiber and lean proteins.

People often complain of other symptoms that are likely to be related to diet as well. Headaches, irritability, laziness, sluggishness, muscle aches and lack of interest in romantic encounters could all be due to poor eating habits. Almost immediately after eating a healthy meal people become more energetic and have an enhanced mental clarity. Within a few days this positive mental outlook leads to the desire to exercise and become more active. Healthy eating has tons of benefits to the mind and body which is why superfoods have become such a popular concept in recent years.

Superfoods That Accelerate Weight Loss

In addition to the health benefits listed above, specific superfoods can be used to regulate digestive functions and the overall metabolism. These two improvements alone will help an individual shed unwanted pounds, but there are even more possibilities to be found inside a few key superfoods. As noted in chapter 4, most Superfoods are rich in antioxidants which remove harmful toxins from the body and reduce inflammatory disorders ranging from acne to arthritis.

People who are trying to lose weight should consider adding these superfoods to their diet:

Hot Peppers – in general, peppers have a variety of health benefits. They can reduce fever and headaches and reduce the inflammation associated with arthritis and other chronic conditions. The active ingredient capsaicin is found in every variety of pepper whether they are hot or sweet. Hot peppers have a special quality in that they provide energy and are natural appetite suppressants that can be easily added to any meal, soup or stew. They can even be eaten as a healthy snack choice.

Nuts and Seeds – high in protein and amino acids but low in sugar and fat, these gems should be staples in every diet. Both of these superfoods will assist with improving digestive and heart health. Nuts in particular have been linked with reducing and regulating blood glucose levels. They are also high in omega-3 fatty acids which reduce harmful cholesterol levels. Along with all of these benefits, nuts and seeds are also naturally high in protein which makes them filling snacks that provide energy and a way to combat feelings of afternoon fatigue.

Beans and Lentils – make great supplements to any diet, including vegetarian meal plans. They are low in fat and calories but provide a more than adequate supply of proteins, fiber, and complex carbohydrates. Beans are a necessity for anyone who is attempting to reduce the risk of diabetes because they absorb slowly into the blood stream and supply the body with only useful ingredients that aid the digestive process. They are great additions for people who struggle with snacking between meals because they are so filling that they prevent hunger pangs for several hours after consumption.

Eggs – despite the brief but negative reputation for having cholesterol laden yolks, eggs are actually great ways to help accelerate weight loss. Because they are high in protein they prevent hunger and subsequent cravings for pastries and other simple carbohydrates. They can be prepared in any number of ways and pair well with most vegetables.

Salmon – all fish contain lean proteins but wild caught Salmon contains the most omega-3 fatty acids when compared pound for pound against other fish and lean meats. It is not only heart healthy but the protein also prevents hunger between meals and regulates insulin sensitivity in the bloodstream. These qualities specifically reduce belly fat and promote the development of healthy lean muscle which then feeds on stored fat throughout the body.

Chapter 6 - Superfoods That Help To Build Muscle

Increasing muscle mass is an integral part of any good fitness regimen. More muscle mass improves BMI, gives you more energy and endurance, burns more fat, and increases overall attractiveness. You may be exercising like a madwoman or a madman, but did you know that diet is just as important to increasing muscle mas as exercise is? It is vital to ensure that the body is given plenty of healthy proteins, fats, vitamins and minerals to rebuild muscle that is worked while exercising to make it even stronger than before. So, which foods are the best to help you build more muscle more quickly? This article will highlight some of the top superfoods to helping you recover from your workouts and increase your muscle mass.

Eggs

Eggs are a solid source of both protein and healthy fats. Many people are concerned about the high amounts of cholesterol in the yolks of eggs. However, cholesterol in eggs shouldn't be a problem as long as they are consumed in moderation. Additionally, dietary cholesterol (the type of cholesterol found in eggs) is unrelated to rates of blood cholesterol, which is the type of cholesterol that can be dangerous if it is too prevalent in the body. Eggs are an excellent economic choice and are incredibly diverse.

Red Meat

Red meat is a jackpot of both protein and nutrients. It is chock full of B vitamins, zinc, and other important vitamins and minerals. High quality cuts of meat can provide healthy fats in good proportions as well as the best flavor.

Nuts

Nuts are a great snack for at home or on the go when you need a big punch of energy that can fit in the palm of your hand. Nuts provide great fats and a lot of protein and also include a good amount of fiber. The best nuts for your health are almonds, pistachios, cashews, walnuts, and Brazil nuts. If you prefer to eat your nuts in mixes, look for products that contain mostly these nuts without much sodium. Unsalted, unflavored nuts are the best option.

Carrots

Carrots pack a big punch of fiber and copious amounts of Vitamin A which are integral to a healthy and strong body. They are easy to eat and are a low calorie snack to pack on the go.

Cottage Cheese

Cottage cheese is the best dairy product for your overall health as well as your muscles. Cottage cheese is loaded with protein, and unlike most other dairy products, isn't laden with fat. Cottage cheese can be eaten plain, or substituted for fats and other less healthy dairy products in many recipes.

Salmon

Salmon is one of the best foods for Omega-3s which can help lower body fat. Additionally, it provides high amounts of protein and is a good source of other vitamins.

Green Tea

Green tea provides a whole host of benefits. Green tea provides a good deal of natural antioxidants and can also function as an aid to digestion that can help regulate and assist in digestion.

Avocado

Avocados are excellent healthy fats that will help satisfy hunger, leading to lower calories and higher quality diet. Avocados are a diverse food that can add flavor and pizzazz to many a dish. Avocados are loaded with vital nutrients.

Olive Oil

Olive Oil is another healthy fat that will help suppress hunger and provide adequate amounts of nutrients to keep the body strong and set the conditions for the body to rapidly build muscle. Olive oil is a great fat to cook with and can be used in place of other oils, butter, and margarine.

Quinoa

This super grain is gluten free and high in both protein and fiber. Quinoa is a healthier alternative to more prevalent grains like rice and flours. Quinoa is versatile and can be eaten hot or cold.

Berries

Berries have one of the highest concentrations of antioxidants which provide a wide array of benefits including strengthening the immune system and helping prevent a multitude of diseases as well as help make the body look and feel younger and more energized.

Spinach

Spinach is one of the best sources of alkaline. Alkaline is a substance that helps strengthen bones and also helps sustain muscle mass. Spinach can be thrown into any smoothie recipe for a nutrient boost. Calcium, magnesium, and zinc are also prominent in the super vegetable.

Turkey

Turkey is incredibly low in fat and high in protein with good amounts of fiber. Turkey is a tasty meat that provides the body with a great deal of some of the leanest meat that can be found. Be sure to eat white turkey meat as the darker variety is much higher in fat and less beneficial for the body.

Oats

Oats are a great grain and an excellent breakfast alternative to most processed cereals and breads. Oats provide healthy, complex carbohydrate that is high in fiber. When paired with proteins and fresh fruits or vegetables, oats can be a killer post workout meal.

Apples

The old adage, "an apple a day keeps the doctor away" holds true when it comes to building muscle mass, too. Apples are known to help increase the body's satisfaction and can help keep you full for longer. Apples boast high amounts of important vitamins and minerals and are easy to incorporate into any lifestyle. Not only can they be added to a variety of dishes, but they can be eaten raw and on the go with ease.

Chapter 7 - Superfoods - Frequently Asked Questions

Many people are wondering what all the fuss about superfoods is about today. In case you are one of them, read some frequently asked questions below to find out more about these foods.

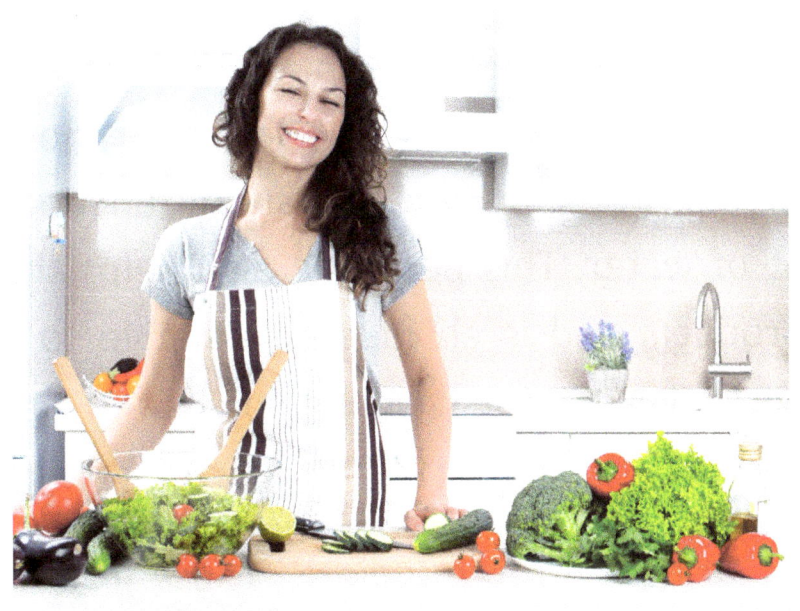

Why are some foods called Superfoods?

Superfoods contain more phytochemicals than other foods. These provide various health benefits. These foods are also is an excellent source of protein, antioxidants and various macronutrients. Superfoods also help the body improve its functioning through their unique features.

Will a supplement provide you the same benefits?

Supplements do not provide the same type of nutrition as Superfoods do. These contain many more things for the body than can be placed into a supplement. The nutrients provided through these foods all work together in a way that is natural for the body to assimilate easily.

Are there any beverages that are considered Superfoods?

Water is the number one beverage that is considered a superfood because of what it does for the body. This clear, no-calorie liquid hydrates every cell in the body. Cells cannot function without the right amount of water. This beverage also helps the body flush out waste products and is an ideal alternative to sugary high-calories drinks that can cause weight gain.

Tea is another beverage in this category. Any type of tea contains antioxidants that fight off free radicals. These free radicals cause the body to become ill with a variety of diseases. Green tea has the most antioxidants since the tea leaves go through less processing than the other leaves used in other types of tea.

What are some Common Superfoods?

Kidney, red, pinto and other types of beans provide the body with insoluble fiber, protein and carbohydrates. They also are a great source for calcium and iron. These can be used in place of meat for a lean protein. Vegetarians often turn to these to make sure they get enough protein each day. Calorie-wise, beans are no higher in calories than meat is. The insoluble fiber helps the body digest food and remove waste products.

Salmon is a fish that falls into this category of foods. It provides the body with high-quality protein, minerals, vitamins, and omega-3 fatty acids. These fatty acids help to reduce inflammation, lessen the risk of heart disease, and can even help the brain in a variety of ways. Replace meat 2 meals a week with this fish for optimal benefits.

Broccoli is a cruciferous vegetable that is packed with all sorts of nutrition. This vegetable is a valuable source of sulforaphane, which helps lower risk for cancer. There is also some proof that this vegetable can lower blood pressure, reduce heart disease, and help protect the body from the effects of diabetes. Other cruciferous vegetables such as kale, cauliflower, and cabbage fall into the superfood category with broccoli.

Blueberries are another well-known, power-packed food. These berries are high in vitamin C, phytoflavinoids, potassium and antioxidants. This makes them ideal for reducing blood pressure, preventing heart disease, lowering the risk of cancer, and lessening inflammation in the body. Blueberries also provide a healthy dose of daily fiber. This helps lower the level of bad cholesterol in the body. Research has also shown the blueberries could slow down the rate that breast cancer cells grow. These are just some of the superfoods known today. There are many others for you to explore.

Does it matter how I prepare the Superfoods for eating?

Yes, it does matter how you prepare these foods for eating. This is because you can damage part of their benefits by adding fats, too much salt, or sugar to them. Many of the foods are ideal fresh and uncooked such as the blueberries, but can also be cooked as long as only healthy ingredients are added to them. Steaming vegetables keep more of the nutrients in them than cooking them to death. Tomatoes are one superfood that improves with cooking. The lycopene increases in tomatoes as they cook and also is easier for the body to assimilate in this state.

How much of the Superfoods do I need to add to my daily diet?

Portion amounts depend on how many total calories you need in a day along with the category of foods about which you are talking. The recommendation for cruciferous vegetables today is that they should take up half your plate. One cup of dry beans cooked provides the body with 16 grams protein. Eight ounces of lean meat on the other hand provides the body with 21 grams protein. This allows you to figure your portions. You need to look up the recommended amounts for each superfood you use.

Are the Superfoods better in organic form?

The organic form of superfoods is better for the body because it eliminates the pesticides and other chemicals used in the traditional growing methods. In addition, non-GMO (genetically modified) versions of these foods have not been altered from their original form. This means that the foods are in their purest form. However, if organic and non-GMO forms of these foods are not readily available to you, then buy the highest quality traditionally produced foods you can.

Are these Superfoods worth eating?

This is not an answer for me to give you. Add them to your diet and prove to yourself the benefits your body will receive. I can testify that they have helped me stay healthier and stronger.

About The Author

Mark Wilson would never ever say that he was a healthy eater since he left his parents home but he can without a doubt say that he found the path back to healthy eating when he realized that he was becoming too addicted to junk foods. He remembered what his parents would say to him as a child that he needed to eat up his vegetables and he would grow up healthy and strong.

When he started to do his research to find out what foods were best for him to eat, he came upon a list of superfoods. This captured his interest and caused him to do even more research on these superfoods before he decided to try them for himself. The success that he had from eating superfoods led him to write his book highlighting the benefits.

www.ingramcontent.com/pod-product-compliance
Ingram Content Group UK Ltd.
Pitfield, Milton Keynes, MK11 3LW, UK
UKHW050419240426
12048UKWH00014B/714